JL BROWN

The Intermittent Fasting Lifestyle

A Quick Guide to Weight Loss, Healing, & A Healthy Life

Contents

1

Introduction

Intermittent Fasting should be viewed as a LIFESTYLE and not just another fad diet. Diets fail, period. However, a few simple changes in the timing of when you eat can ultimately change your life and your overall health for good! Some of these methods may seem extreme, but there are plenty of methods to intermittent fasting and my goal with this book is to help you find the method that works best for you so you can start your journey to a longer, healthier life.

So what is Intermittent Fasting? Intermittent fasting is a popular dietary approach that involves cycling between periods of fasting and eating. It has gained attention for its health benefits and effectiveness in weight management.

The concept of intermittent fasting is not focused on what you eat, but rather on when you eat. There are many different intermittent fasting options, which will be covered in more detail within the book. However, the most common ones are:

- **Time-Restricted Fasting**
- **Alternate-Day Fasting**
- **Eat Stop Eat**
- **The Warrior Diet**

The primary goal of intermittent fasting is to extend the period your body spends in a fasted state. During fasting periods, your body depletes glycogen stores for energy and begins to rely on stored fat for fuel, which can lead to weight loss. Intermittent fasting offers numerous benefits, including:

- **Weight Loss**: By eating fewer meals, intermittent fasting can lead to an automatic reduction in calorie intake. Additionally, it can increase metabolism during the fasting periods.
- **Insulin Resistance**: Intermittent Fasting may improve insulin sensitivity, potentially reducing the risk of type 2 diabetes.
- **Heart Health**: Intermittent Fasting could improve various risk factors for heart disease such as blood pressure, cholesterol levels, triglycerides, and inflammatory markers.
- **Brain Health**: Intermittent Fasting increases the brain hormone BDNF and may aid the growth of new nerve cells. It might also protect against Alzheimer's disease.
- **Cancer Prevention**: Animal studies suggest that intermittent fasting may help prevent cancer.
- **Anti-Aging**: Intermittent Fasting can extend lifespan in rats. Studies showed that fasted rats lived longer than the non-fasted ones.

It's essential to note that intermittent fasting is not suitable for everyone, particularly those with certain medical conditions or individuals who are pregnant, breastfeeding, or have a history of eating disorders. It's recommended to consult with a healthcare professional or registered dietitian before starting any fasting regimen.

Intermittent fasting is a tool that can be effective for weight loss and health improvement, but it's important to approach it sensibly and choose a method that is sustainable for your lifestyle. It's also vital to focus on nutritious foods during the eating periods for overall health.

2

How Intermittent Fasting Works

Understanding some of the in's and out's of intermittent fasting is important so you don't feel like you're just starving yourself for weight loss as there is so much more to it than shedding some pounds. Obviously many start intermittent fasting for that reason, but the additional benefits to your overall health can be life changing. While in a fasted state, your body will first use up any remaining nutritive stores within the digestive tract for energy. Once these stores have been depleted, your body will turn to the fat reserves for its next source of energy which can lead to weight loss. As an added bonus, while in this fasted state, your tissues and organs are primed for repair as cells undergo renovation, and other forms of healing can happen within the body.

Changes in Hormones & Metabolism

The levels of Human Growth Hormone (HGH) can increase as much as five fold during intermittent fasting. Higher levels of HGH facilitate fat burning and muscle gain; however, HGH's importance extends beyond what many realize. As we age, the pituitary gland reduces HGH production, which can lead to weakening muscles and bones over time. HGH is also crucial for brain function, helping to alleviate brain fog and increasing alertness and motivation. Furthermore, it aids in improving memory and cognitive function. Based on my experience with intermittent fasting, I feel most focused and energized during the final few hours before my fasting period concludes.

During fasting periods, the body undergoes a number of changes at a cellular and molecular level. Short-term fasting actually increases your metabolic rate by 3.6-14%, helping you burn even more calories. As you become more familiar with fasting and can push your fast to the 16:8 method, your body can turn into a fat burning machine as there is a higher level of glycogen stores being depleted.

Cellular Repair and Autophagy

When fasted, glucose and insulin levels will decrease which ultimately starves a cell of its nutrition and allows it to initiate cellular repair processes known as autophagy. Autophagy (pronounced "ah-TAH-fah-gee") is the body's process where cells digest and remove old and dysfunctional proteins that build up inside cells.. These "recycled" parts are then turned into Amino Acids and used for energy. As with many changes in our bodies as we age, autophagy is another process that slows which in some studies, may be associated with diseases such as, Cancer, Alzheimer's, Parkinson's, Crohn's, heart & liver disease, and diabetes. There is no current proof or evidence that you can prevent any disease by inducing autophagy and in no way am I suggesting that intermittent fasting is the cure for any disease. Autophagy is just another positive benefit that can happen while intermittent fasting.

3

Health Benefits of Intermittent Fasting

We've touched on a few of the benefits related to hormones and metabolism, but let's dive into more of the benefits that come along with intermittent fasting.

Weight Management and Fat Loss

When most people start their intermittent fasting journey, it is often with the goal of shedding unwanted weight. This method allows individuals to focus on when they eat rather than being overly restrictive about what they eat. Diets are notorious for their high failure rates, partially because the requirement to eliminate all enjoyable foods makes adherence challenging. While intermittent fasting does not necessitate cutting out everything you enjoy, it is still important to consume all the proper proteins and nutrients that constitute a healthy diet.

Ketosis is a metabolic state in which your body burns fat for energy instead of carbohydrates. Many individuals who practice fasting naturally enter ketosis during their fasting period. Depending on the types of food consumed, it is possible to remain in a state of ketosis, continuing to burn fat.

Ghrelin, often referred to as the 'hunger hormone,' is commonly thought to increase significantly during fasting—leading to heightened appetite. However, some research suggests that fasting may, conversely, decrease ghrelin production, which could, over time, lead to a lessened appetite.

Adopting intermittent fasting as more than a temporary diet but as a lifestyle can lead to sustained weight loss, helping you achieve and maintain a healthy weight.

Improved Insulin Sensitivity

Fasting prompts a significant drop in insulin levels, which in turn facilitates fat burning. This decrease makes stored body fat more accessible as a source of energy. Additionally, fasting can lead to reductions in LDL cholesterol, blood triglycerides, inflammatory markers, blood sugar, and insulin resistance, all of which contribute to a lower risk of heart disease.

According to the National Library of Medicine, research has shown that intermittent fasting diets exert therapeutic effects on blood glucose and lipids in patients with metabolic syndrome and significantly improve insulin sensitivity. As such, intermittent fasting may be considered an adjunct treatment strategy for preventing the onset and progression of chronic diseases.

Reduced Inflammation

Inflammation in the body is a common culprit behind pain. Those suffering from joint or back pain could really benefit from intermittent fasting as it helps reduce inflammation and allows the body to heal. I personally have grappled with back pain due to an injury to my L5-S1 disc caused by improper exercise form. The injury resulted in nearly a year of chronic back and leg pain. While chiropractic care and physical therapy offered some relief, the pain persistently lingered. Around the time the Keto Diet began garnering widespread attention, I started exploring intermittent fasting. I recall listening to a podcast where the guest discussed his daily regimen and how he incorporated Keto with intermittent fasting, reaping a broader spectrum of health benefits beyond just weight loss. This piqued my interest.

After extensive research and reading about the numerous benefits—reduced inflammation being one of them—I decided that intermittent fasting was something I needed to try. That was roughly eight years ago, and I haven't looked back since. The pain in my back has dissipated, and I credit much of this improvement to the decreased inflammation in my body. However, I must clarify that this was my experience and it may not reflect everyone's journey with intermittent fasting. If you're dealing with chronic pain, it's essential to consult with a physician and discuss whether intermittent fasting is appropriate for you. I prefer natural solutions that allow my body to heal itself over medication when feasible, so for me, the decision to try intermittent fasting was an easy one.

Potential Anti-Aging

The largest organ of our body is our skin, and as we age, it is often one of the first to show signs of aging. Fasting can accelerate the repair of tissues and organs beyond what is achieved through eating a healthy diet alone. During fasting, cells undergo autophagy, which rejuvenates them—including those within the skin—resulting in a more youthful and improved skin appearance. The increased circulation that comes with weight loss and reduced inflammation can also contribute to diminishing fine lines, blotches, and blemishes that often accompany aging.

4

Potential Risks and Considerations

While IF has grown in popularity among those seeking weight loss and other health benefits, it's crucial to recognize that this lifestyle change may not suit everyone. Understanding the potential risks is essential to ensure that this practice will be beneficial for you.

Nutritional Considerations

Transitioning to an intermittent fasting lifestyle requires careful nutritional planning. During eating windows, it is essential to consume a balanced diet rich in all necessary macro- and micronutrients to maintain health and bodily functions. The compressed eating periods should not be seen as a green light to indulge indiscriminately; they are an opportunity to nourish the body mindfully.

Individuals must ensure they receive adequate vitamins, minerals, and fiber—key components for digestive health, immune function, and overall well-being. Emphasizing nutrient-dense foods, such as whole grains, proteins, healthy fats, fruits, and vegetables, is crucial. Otherwise, there's a risk of developing nutritional deficiencies, which can lead to health issues like anemia, osteoporosis, and electrolyte imbalances.

Impact on Energy Levels and Performance

Energy levels and overall performance can be significantly impacted by IF. Some individuals report heightened mental clarity and energy after adapting to fasting routines, likely due to the body's shift to fat as a fuel source after glycogen stores are depleted. However, others may experience lethargy, decreased concentration, and reduced exercise performance, particularly during the adjustment phase.

Physical performance may also be affected by when the eating window aligns with exercise routines. Exercising in a fasted state might not provide the immediate energy needed for high-intensity activities, leading to quicker exhaustion. In contrast, exercising within the eating window can contribute to more stable and sustained energy output.

Potential Negative Effects

Though many adapt well to intermittent fasting, potential downsides may still exist, including:

- Hunger and irritability, often referred to as "hangry" states, especially during adaptation.
- Potential for overeating or unhealthy eating during feeding windows due to extreme hunger.
- Disrupted social eating patterns, which can affect social relationships and work schedules.
- Potential to exacerbate disordered eating behaviors, particularly in individuals prone to eating disorders.
- One of the more subtle risks is the potential for underestimating

the importance of meal timing and composition, which can lead to metabolic disruptions and other health issues.

Precautions for Specific Medical Conditions

While IF has been associated with health benefits like improved insulin sensitivity and weight reduction, caution is advised for those with or susceptible to certain medical conditions:

- Diabetes: Patients, especially those on insulin or other glucose-lowering medications, should carefully monitor their blood sugar levels as IF can significantly alter insulin requirements and cause hypoglycemia.
- Heart Disease: Individuals with cardiovascular issues should consult with a healthcare professional, as altering meal times can impact blood pressure and heart rate.
- Women's Health: Women, particularly those with a history of fertility issues or irregular menstrual cycles, should be cautious as IF can affect reproductive hormones.
- Moreover, individuals with a history of eating disorders should avoid IF, as the cycles of fasting and feasting could trigger unhealthy behaviors.

In conclusion, while IF may offer several potential health benefits, it is incumbent upon each individual to carefully assess their health status, nutritional needs, lifestyle, and any specific medical concerns before embarking on such a regimen. Consulting with healthcare providers for personalized advice is always the best course of action when considering changes to one's diet, particularly for those with pre-existing health conditions. With careful planning and monitoring, intermittent fasting can be integrated into one's lifestyle, potentially offering an array of benefits without compromising nutritional health and well-being.

5

Different Methods of Intermittent Fasting

12/12 Method - The 12/12 method is the most popular for beginners. This IF method means you would fast for 12 hours then have an eating window for 12 hours. The majority of your fasting happens while you are asleep which makes this option more appealing and easier to stick to. For example: If you eat your last meal of the day at 7:00 pm then you would wait until 7:00 AM the following day to eat again. Once you have succeeded at the 12/12 method, try pushing your fasting time an additional hour every few days until you reach the 16/8 method.

16/8 Method - The 16/8 method is more intermediate, and suggested after you have mastered the 12/12 method. With this method, you will fast for 16 hours and have an 8 hour window for eating. For example: If you finish your last meal of the day at 7:00 PM then you would wait until 11:00 AM the next day. This method is where you can really see your body begin to change as many of the benefits from fasting come when you are in a fasted state for longer periods of time.

5:2 Method - The 5:2 method means you eat for five days per week, but don't really have to think about restricting calories. Then on the other two days, you reduce your calorie intake to a quarter of your daily needs. This is about 500 calories per day for women, and 600 for men. You can choose whichever two days of the week you prefer, as long as there is at least one non-fasting day in between them. One common way of planning the week is to fast on Mondays and Thursdays, with two or three small meals, then eat normally/healthy for the rest of the week.

Alternate Day Fasting - Alternate day intermittent fasting is a pattern of eating that alternates periods of fasting with periods of eating. This type of IF typically involves a cycle where you eat normally one day and then either completely fast or significantly restrict your caloric intake (typically around 500 calories) the next day.

Here's a basic overview of how alternate day fasting might look:

- Fasting Days: On fasting days, you consume very few calories. Some variations allow for up to 500 calories, while others recommend a full fast with no caloric intake. The idea is to create a significant caloric deficit to promote weight loss and potentially trigger other health benefits.

-

- Feeding Days: On feeding days, you return to eating normally. It's important to eat a well-balanced diet on these days so that your body gets the nutrients it needs to function properly. It's discouraged to overeat or binge on feeding days, as this can counteract the benefits of the fasting days.

Eat-Stop-Eat Method - This method involves 24-hour fasts once or twice per week. During the fasting periods, you consume no calories, although you are allowed to drink calorie-free beverages like water, tea, and black coffee. After the 24-hour fasting period, you return to eating normally until the next fasting period begins.

Here's how the Eat Stop Eat method typically works.

- Choose Your Fasting Days: Pick one or two days per week to conduct your 24-hour fast. It's often recommended that you do not do them consecutively to help manage and better distribute your energy levels throughout the week.

- Start Fasting: Begin your fast at a convenient time. For example, if you finish dinner at 7 p.m., you would not eat again until 7 p.m. the following day. I would recommend finishing your last meal between the times of 5 - 7:00 pm.

- Break the Fast Gently: When you complete the 24-hour fasting period, you should aim to eat a normal-sized meal, not larger than usual, to avoid overeating.

20/4 also known as the Warrior Diet - The Warrior Diet is a form of intermittent fasting popularized by Ori Hofmekler in the early 2000s. It's based on the idea that ancient warriors thrived on a diet of infrequent, but large meals. The eating pattern involves a cycle of lengthy periods of undereating or fasting during the day, followed by a short period of overeating at night.

Here's how the Warrior Diet typically works:

- Fasting Phase (20 hours): During the day, one undertakes a fasting-phase that lasts for about 20 hours. During this period, you're encouraged to consume small amounts of dairy products, hard-boiled eggs, raw fruits, and vegetables, as well as plenty of fluids. The idea is to keep calorie intake to a minimum.

- Eating Window (4 hours): The fasting phase is followed by a 4-hour eating window in the evening. This window is when the majority of daily calorie intake should occur. During this period, you can eat one large meal or multiple small meals, and there are fewer restrictions on the types of food you can eat.

- The diet promotes the consumption of whole, unprocessed foods during the overeating phase and emphasizes the importance of listening to your body's hunger signals.

Of all the fasting methods listed above, the 16/8 method is the one I have practiced for many years. I began with the 12/12 method and gradually increased my fast an hour at a time until I reached the 16 hour mark. I have seen great results with this method and have made it my daily routine. It no longer feels like fasting, but rather just my typical day. It's definitely a lifestyle now and one I don't see foresee changing.

6

Getting Started with Intermittent Fasting

Let's dive into how to get started on your Intermittent Fasting journey. One thing to consider if you are wanting to lose weight is how many calories and macronutrients you should be getting each day. There are various ways to determine how to calculate your calorie intake, such as different apps available for download on your phone or do a quick internet search for "calorie calculator" where you'll find the free calculator on calculator.net. Here you'll enter your age, gender, height & weight and how active you are during the day and it will calculate your calories as well as your macros (protein, carbs, fats, & sugars). This calculator can help you with your calories for maintaining or losing weight. Once you know how many calories you should be getting each day, you can start to come up with a plan.

Setting Your Fasting Schedule

When beginning Intermittent Fasting for the first time, it is important that you start with an easy fast. For beginners, I would suggest using the 12/12 method. This is the easiest to start with. It is important to get your body used to fasting before choosing a method so you do not set yourself up for failure. Remember IF is a lifestyle and not a diet so start easy and work your way up to a longer time of fasting as there are many benefits to each option.

Tips for a Successful Intermittent Fasting Journey

- **Be Prepared**! Being prepared is, hands down, the most crucial part of a successful IF journey. If you are not equipped with nutritious foods on hand, you'll be more likely to reach for the wrong kinds of food when your fasting period ends. Like any weight loss program, it's imperative to fuel your body with nutritious food if you expect to see any positive change. If your goal is to lose weight, you also need to assess how many calories your body needs to consume to maintain a caloric deficit. Meal prepping can be incredibly helpful and keep you on track. Try preparing a week's worth of lunches and have dinner plans ready so that you know exactly what you'll be cooking. Failing to have meals planned may tempt you to eat out, which, while fine occasionally, can hinder your progress if you have a specific goal in mind. Eating at home is usually a healthier choice.

- Track Your Food. As you begin your IF journey, one of the most effective ways to ensure you're getting the right amount of nutrients is by tracking your food. You can keep a food journal to note what you're eating each day, or you can use one of the various apps available for your phone that simplify the process. Most of these apps come with barcode scanners that let you quickly log the nutritional content of packaged foods. They can also help you determine the calorie content of fresh foods like fruits and vegetables, which typically don't come with nutrition labels. If you're new to food journaling, you might be surprised to discover how much or how little you're actually consuming. It's vital to ensure you're getting adequate amounts of protein, healthy fats, and carbohydrates (yes, carbs—they aren't the enemy) each day for the most effective IF experience possible.

- Stay Hydrated. Your body requires extra hydration when fasting because low levels of insulin lead to slight dehydration. Make sure you consume an adequate amount of liquids to maintain your water balance to prevent dehydration.Drinking water might trick your mind when you are hungry and help with food cravings. If you don't stay hydrated, you may end up overeating when your fasting period ends, which will produce no results from your efforts, and could potentially lead to additional weight gain.

- Being hungry when fasting is absolutely normal. Tea and black coffee are allowed for almost any fasting protocol. Tea (especially green tea) and coffee don't just have important antioxidants to fight inflammation in the body, but they also have natural hunger suppressant components. Having a cup of tea or coffee significantly lowers hunger and stomach growling. Keep in mind that these drinks are diuretics, meaning they increase the excretion of water and minerals through excessive urination. After every cup of tea or coffee you should drink a glass of water (with a dash of salt) to keep your water-electrolytes equilibrium.

- Good quality sleep is essential when you fast. Lack of sleep puts your body in a stressed state, where your adrenal glands produce cortisol. This hormone affects not only your mood in a negative way but also your insulin levels, which rise even without eating. Poor sleep decreases the beneficial effects of fasting and makes you hungry, and can promote sugar cravings.

- Keep yourself busy. One of the best ways to get through the fasting period is to keep yourself busy. For most fasting schedules, you'll be sleeping through much of your fasting period, but for the remaining time, it's good to keep your mind occupied. By keeping yourself busy you will be able to ignore your feelings of hunger. For me, I like to stay as busy as possible and if I feel the hunger knocking, I will drink water or maybe another cup of coffee to push through.

Another great tip is to exercise while fasting as it will help keep your mind and body busy. As a beginner at fasting, you may want to wait until after you have broken your fast to exercise as it may make you feel more hungry if you're not used to exercising on an empty stomach. If you are someone who needs a pre-workout or like to take BCAA's while working out, you will need to wait until you are no longer in your fasting period as both types of supplements will break your fast.

- Be sure to get in your allotted calories throughout your eating window. This will significantly help the next day during your fasting period. By consuming too little calories, you will feel hungry sooner and you may be tempted to break your fast too soon. If you are consuming less than 1200 calories in a day, you may be causing more harm to your body than you may think. Long term restricted calories will lead to bone and muscle loss and your metabolism will slow. This is not healthy or sustainable in the long term and definitely not recommended for anyone trying to better their overall health.

- When it comes time to break your fast it is important that you are not breaking your fast with junk food, but instead breaking it with proteins or fruits and vegetables. Your body will crave whatever food you choose to break your fast with. There are conflicting opinions on what will break your fast. Some believe a single calorie will break your fast while others say as long as you stay under 50 calories, your body is still in a fasted state.

- I am a coffee drinker and I like to add a bit of heavy cream to my coffee. I add only enough to keep it under 50 calories and I still see the benefits of IF. If you are one who likes straight black coffee, more power to you and you are free to drink your coffee in the morning without breaking your fast. However, if you're like me and just can't do black coffee, and you are not seeing any results, I would suggest drinking water until your fast is over, then consume your coffee.

Common Challenges and How to Overcome Them

- Hunger and cravings - This is the most common side effect of intermittent fasting. When you first begin IF you will experience hunger; that's just something to expect if you've never fasted before. This side effect usually takes about 4-21 days for your body to get used to being in a fasted state. It is best to use the tips that we listed to help you push through your fasting experience.

- Headaches can occur when staring IF. This can be common at the beginning of the IF process as some may experience the side effects from caffeine and sugar withdrawal. "Fasting Headaches" are usually located in the frontal region of the brain and tend to be more mild than heavy. Most can expect that the headache symptoms usually go away around the first week of IF. For those that experience headaches more often, you may want to start slow with IF, such as the 12/12 method to see how your body reacts. Diving into a more intermediate method may trigger unwanted and unnecessary headaches.

- It is possible that digestive issues may occur as a result of dietary changes. When making significant changes to your diet, some individuals may experience symptoms such as gas, bloating, or diarrhea initially. It's important to note that not all side effects will be negative. For instance, if you're incorporating more vegetables and grains into your diet compared to before, experiencing short-term digestive issues is a common adaptation process for your body.

- Fatigue and low energy can be common if you don't stay hydrated and you don't get enough sleep. For some, low blood sugar levels can also make you feel tired and weak, this is why it's imperative that you consume your full amount of allotted calories during your eating periods. As your body adjusts to fasting periods, fatigue should no longer be an issue and you should actually start to feel more energized and focused.

- Dehydration is something to be very aware of while fasting. As one begins fasting, the body can release large amounts of water and salt in urine. This process is known as natural diuresis or natriuresis of fasting. Whether fasting or not, you should consume half your bodyweight in ounces of water each day. So if you weigh 200 lbs, you should be drinking 100oz of water each day. Adding a few drops of trace minerals or a pinch of high quality sea salt to your water will provide your body with the natural minerals it needs and will help replenish lost electrolytes. It may not sound so appealing to add salt to water, but if you add just a pinch, you really don't taste it.

7

Frequently Asked Questions

Below we'll cover some of the commonly asked questions related to intermittent fasting. While you may have additional questions, these should cover the basics.

Can I drink liquids during the fast?

Yes. Water should become your best friend during your fasting periods. Black coffee, and unsweetened tea are fine too. Do not add sugar or any flavor additives, even if they say zero calorie, to any of your beverages. As mentioned before, there are some who say less than 50 calories will keep you in a fasted state, so milk or cream can be added to your coffee as long as you don't add too much. Coffee can be particularly beneficial during a fast, especially in the beginning as it can help curb your appetite until your fast is over.

Can I take supplements while working out?

It's okay to take regular vitamin pills and capsules while fasting, as they are unlikely to affect insulin levels, but vitamins and supplements sold as gummies, liquids, or chewable tablets are typically sweetened and can stimulate an insulin response, so, if you use these, take them during your eating window.

Here is a list of supplements that will break your fast as they will spike your insulin levels due to the calories or ingredients they have in them. Many may contain zero calories, however because of the ingredients, they can cause your insulin to rise and pull you out of a fasted state.

1. Protein
2. Gummy Vitamins/Coated Supplements
3. Bone Broth
4. Collagen
5. MCT Oil
6. Branched-Chain Amino Acids (BCAAs)
7. Pre Workout supplements

Will Intermittent Fasting cause muscle loss?

All weight loss methods can cause muscle loss if you are not actively working out, which is why it's important to incorporate strength training, such as weight lifting and keep your protein intake high. Ladies, it's important to note that you will NOT bulk up by lifting moderate weight. Your body needs muscle and it's very much needed to support overall health as you age. No one is saying you need to lift like a bodybuilder, but don't be afraid to pick up a few dumbbells during your workouts.

Will Intermittent Fasting slow down my metabolism?

No. Older studies show that short-term fasts actually boost metabolism. However, longer fasts of 3 or more days can suppress metabolism. This is why it's crucial to make sure you are consuming all your allotted calories during your eating window. If you don't eat enough, then yes, your metabolism can slow.

8

Final Thoughts

There are many health and weight loss benefits to intermittent fasting that, to me, make it one of the best lifestyle changes one can make—at least that's been my experience. I have never thought of IF as a diet since diets are hard to stick with and restrict what you can and can't eat. If you're starting IF primarily for weight loss, you probably shouldn't reach for junk food, as you still want to ensure you're maintaining a caloric deficit to lose weight. However, when you feel the need to have that slice of pizza or that piece of cake for your birthday, go ahead! I'm not saying you should eat the whole pizza or more than a single piece of cake, but when you're managing your calories in other ways, indulging once in a while is okay. Just don't make it a daily habit, and you should still witness the benefits of IF.

As you've probably noticed throughout this book, I'm pretty partial to the 16/8 method. As I mentioned before, it's something I've practiced for years, so it feels normal now, and I don't feel like I'm fasting. I still enjoy food and don't restrict myself or feel like I'm dieting. I'm content with my weight and have learned how much I need to eat to take in the necessary protein and other macronutrients my body requires.

If you are considering adopting any of these methods, I would recommend choosing one that fits your lifestyle and committing to it for a minimum of 30 days. If you find after 30 days that you're not noticing any changes or seeing results, perhaps try a different method to determine if it's more effective for you. Consistency is key with IF, and once you find your rhythm, it genuinely will become part of your lifestyle, and you won't even realize you're fasting each day.

I wish you the best of luck on your intermittent fasting journey and hope you'll discover how it can become more than a diet but a sustainable lifestyle. Take it one day at a time, and be patient with the results. Remember, consistency is key, and if you stick with it and remain focused on your goals, I am confident you will see the transformative effects on your health and body.

If you found this book helpful, I'd be very appreciative if you left a favorable review for the book on Amazon.

9

Resources

Intermittent Fasting: What is it, and how does it work? (2023, September 29). Johns Hopkins Medicine. https://www.hopkinsmedicine.org/health/wellness-and-prevention/intermittent-fasting-what-is-it-and-how-does-it-work

Moore, M. D. (n.d.). Fasting can heal the human organism of disease and reverse the aging process. https://www.alliedacademies.org/articles/fasting-can-heal-the-human-organism-of-disease-and-reverse-the-ageing-process-11647.html#:~:text=Tissues%20and%20organs%20are%20repaired,also%20seen%20during%20a%20fast.

Hayes, K., RN. (2023, November 7). What is autophagy? Verywell Health. https://www.verywellhealth.com/how-autophagy-works-4210008#:~:text=Autophagy%20is%20a%20process%20that,or%20to%20form%20new%20proteins.

Calorie calculator. (n.d.). https://www.calculator.net/calorie-calculator.html